I0075993

All About
TRANSFERRING
PEOPLE SAFELY

Our thanks to Laura Flynn R.N., B.N., M.B.A. and Sherry Collis, L.P.N., B.B.A. for the development of this book.

Our thanks also to the following organizations: National Pressure Ulcer Advisory Board , Wound Ostomy Continence Nurses members, The Agency for Health Care Policy and the Registered Nurses Association of Ontario for their reference Long Term Care positioning guidelines.

ISBN # 978 1 896616 61 2

© 2013 Mediscript Communications Inc.

Transferring patients. Moving patients in long term care. Moving patients from beds. Patient transfers.

www.mediscript.net

Printed in Canada

Book and Front Cover design by:
Brian Adamson, www.AdamsonGraphics.net

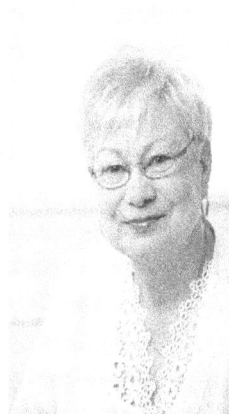

CONTENTS

INTRODUCTION

This book provides basic, non controversial and trusted information that can help a wide spectrum of readers.

The primary objective of the information is to help a person provide effective quality care to a loved one or someone in his or her care.

Transferring someone in your care can be risky both for you and the person being cared for. Consequently, knowing the well-established basics of care and techniques can be invaluable.

All the information is reliable and was written by a group of eminent nurse educators who ensured the information complies with best practice guidelines and satisfies the various accreditation and regulatory bodies. Because there is so much unreliable information on the internet, you can be assured the "all about" publications are HON (Health On the Net) certified.

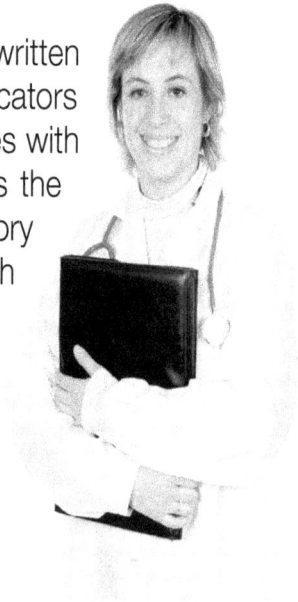

This book can be an invaluable aid to:

- A caregiver caring for a relative or friend
- A health worker seeking a reference aid
- A patient or person needing to be transferred
- Any person involved in health care wishing to expand his or her knowledge

AN IMPORTANT MESSAGE
FROM THE PUBLISHER

Each person's treatment, advice, medical aids, physical therapy and other approaches to health care are unique and highly dependant upon the diagnosis and overall assessment by the medical team.

We emphasize therefore that the information within this book is not a substitute for the advice and treatment from a health care professional.

This book only provides the well accepted generic practices of transferring patients in a health care setting. At facilities such as long term care faciltiies, nursing homes etc. you should always check with the facilty policy prior to any transferring of patients or clients.

With all this in mind, the publishers and authors disclaim any responsibility for any adverse effects resulting directly or indirectly from the suggestions contained within this book or from any misunderstanding of the content on the part of the reader.

HAVE YOU HEARD

Tips for losing weight

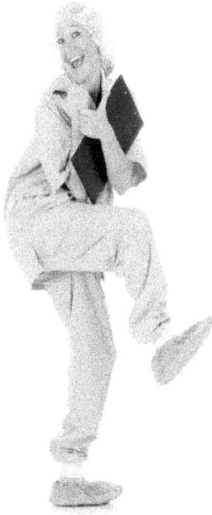

- When weighing, remove everything, including glasses. In this case blurred vision is an asset.

- Never weigh yourself with wet hair.

- Weigh yourself after a haircut; this is good for at least half a pound.

- Use cheap scales only, never the medical kind, because they are always five pounds off...to your advantage, of course.

Source: www.nursefriendly.com

HOW MUCH DO YOU KNOW

It helps at the start of learning about a topic to assess what you know or what attitudes you have about transferring people.

The following questions will provide you with an idea of how knowledgeable you already are about the topic. Just circle the letter to indicate what you think is the best answer and check out the answers on the following page:

1. You are assisting a family member with left-sided weakness into a chair. Where should you place the chair?

a. So the person can move toward her weaker side.

b. So the person can move toward her stronger side.

c. It doesn't matter what side the chair is on.

2. Before transferring the person, you should assess which of the following?

a. Age

b. Hearing and sight

c. Use of alcohol

d. b and c only

e. a, b and c

3. Using good technique during client transfers decreases the chance of injury to the worker and to the person being transfered.

a. True

b. False

4. You are moving the person to a chair. He cannot assist. Is this:

a. A lift

b. A transfer

5. A pull sheet is often referred to as a draw sheet.

a. True

b. False

6. Pivoting means allowing the family member to sit on the side of the bed before standing.

a. True

b. False

7. Both side rails should remain up when moving the person.

a. True

b. False

ANSWERS

1. **a.** Place the chair so the person can move toward her weaker side. This allows her to use the strength available in her stronger side.

2. **b.** The person's hearing and sight are very important for transferring them.

3. **a.** True.

4. **a.** When your family member cannot help at all, this is called a lift.

5. **a.** True. The words "pull sheet" and "draw sheet" are interchangeable.

6. **b.** False. Pivoting means the person's body is turned without touching the spine.

7. **b.** False. Raised side rails provide a greater challenge and make transferring more difficult.

SOMETHING TO THINK ABOUT...

Whatever I have tried to do in my life, I have tried with all my heart to do well.

Charles Dickens

TRANSFERRING PEOPLE SAFELY

Have you ever had back pain due to lifting a family member? Have you ever wondered if there was an easier and safer way of moving the person? If you have, you are not alone. This review will give you information about ways to transfer people as safely as possible, both for you and the person you are caring for.

Transferring and lifting people are the most physically stressful tasks for caregivers. This is important because as a caregiver you may need to transfer and lift your loved one many times during the day. The difference between a transfer and a lift is that the person assists with a transfer, but not with a lift.

Certain factors related to the person and to the situation can cause back pain. Factors related to the person include: his or her weight, inability to bear weight, changes in behavior, and aggressive behavior. Examples of factors related to the situation include: height of the bed, confined workspace, transfer surfaces that are not at the same height, and wheelchairs without adjustable arms. Most caregivers are forced into awkward postures because they must adapt to the needs of the person for whom they are caring.

Of course, not following the principles of keeping your back safe is also a problem. Examples of problems include: improper holding, awkward lifting positions, and frequent stooping and bending.

The technique used during the transfer as well as the weight of the person can significantly increase the risk of injury. Therefore, it is important to use the proper technique. A safe transfer is always the main concern, both for you and your loved one.

SOME WORDS TO KNOW

Dangling - Allowing the person to sit on the edge of the bed for a short period of time before attempting to stand. Dangling prevents the person's blood pressure from dropping quickly as position is changed.

When the person has been in one position for a long period of time, blood tends to stay in the legs. If his position is quickly changed from lying to standing, a decreased blood supply to the brain causes dizziness. People who are taking blood pressure pills or who have not been drinking or eating adequately are at an increased risk. Allowing the person to sit on the side of the bed for a few minutes gives the blood a chance to circulate.

To assist with dangling, put the bed in the lowest position. Have your family member rest her feet on the floor or on a footstool. Encourage her to move her arms, legs, and feet while dangling. Stand in front of her to protect against a forward fall.

Pivoting - A technique used to turn the body without twisting the spine. One foot is positioned ahead of the other. The heels are raised slightly and the entire body is turned on the balls of the feet as one unit, without twisting the back.

Pull sheet - Can also be referred to as a draw sheet, lift sheet, or turn sheet. The sheet is placed under the person's body, from shoulders to thighs, to help with moving or turning.

Weight shift - Involves shifting, or moving, all of your weight from one foot to the other. Weight is shifted in the direction you want to move the person.

GENERAL PRINCIPLES FOR TRANSFERRING SOMEONE

Certain general principles apply to every situation where you must transfer a client or family member. They are very important to the safety of everyone involved.

Assessment

Assessing your loved one will give you valuable information about the level of assistance that will be needed. Knowing this will help you plan the move and will help keep you both safe. You should assess the following:

- age of the person
- level of consciousness and awareness
- ability to follow directions and cooperate
- level of mobility, hearing and sight
- use of alcohol and medications

Plan the move

Make sure you are able to complete the move by yourself. If not, get the assistance you need. Always follow the guidelines for keeping your back safe.

Explain what you are doing

Encourage the client to assist as much as possible. Provide him with eyeglasses if needed. He will be able to assist more and will not become as fearful if he can see. Give him simple, easy directions throughout the transfer. "We are going to stand you up on the count of three."

Maintain privacy

Ensure your family member's privacy is maintained. Keep her covered as much as possible.

Clutter

Ensure the area is uncluttered to guard against tripping. Make sure the floor is dry to prevent slipping. Ensure there is adequate lighting.

Prevent movement

Use the brakes or locks on the wheels of the bed, stretcher, chair, or wheelchair if present. The locks will prevent the bed or chair from moving unexpectedly during the transfer.

Raise the side rail on the side of the bed opposite to the one where you are working (unless there is another caregiver on that side). Make sure that any tubes or lines that are connected to the person (IV lines, catheter bags) are positioned so that they are not in the way and will not be pulled during the move.

If transferring someone into a tub or shower, safety rails and non-skid surfaces should be present. Safety rails near the toilet will help during transfers to and from the toilet.

Comfort

Following the transfer, ensure that your family member is comfortable. Whenever you leave him, arrange necessary items (call bell, water, telephone) within his reach to avoid overreaching.

Leave the bed in its lowest position.

Communicate

If your loved one is uncooperative with particular devices or transfer techniques, explain the reasons for the device or technique. Give her the opportunity to discuss concerns. Perhaps she is afraid. If there is an opportunity for her to make a choice, consider her preferences.

BACK SAFETY

The following is a brief summary of the principles used to keep your back safe. These principles must be maintained during every lift or transfer:

- Do not lift anything, or anyone, that is heavier than 35% of your body weight. For example, if you weigh 150 pounds (68.2 kilograms), the most you should lift is 52.5 pounds (23.8 kilograms). Therefore, if the person is unable to assist, you can only lift a very small person (such as a child) by yourself.

- Maintain a wide base of support. Your feet should be shoulder width apart.

- Stand close to the person who is being moved.

- Bend the knees. Use the legs, not the back, to lift.

- Do not twist as you are lifting.

- Tighten the muscles of your buttocks, stomach, legs and arms to prepare for the move.

- Do not work against gravity.

- Break up a heavy task into small parts, if possible. This is so muscles are not contracted for a prolonged period.

- Avoid overreaching and bending over. If possible, raise or lower the bed to a good height for the task.

EQUIPMENT TO USE DURING TRANSFERS

The use of certain devices can reduce the physical stress of transferring and lifting people.

Transfer belt

A transfer belt provides something around the person's waist that you can grasp to assist with the move. If a transfer belt is not available, a regular belt can be used.

Sling

A regular sling can be used to support a paralyzed arm. An unsupported, paralyzed arm may get injured or may interfere with a safe transfer.

Sliding boards

There are two types of sliding boards that act as a "bridge". A short board is used to move the person from the bed to the chair. A longer board is used to move the person from the bed to a stretcher.

Overhead bar

The overhead bar, or trapeze, is attached to the bed frame. It hangs over the person's upper body. He or she grabs this bar to assist with moving in bed.

Mechanical lift

A mechanical lift is a safe way to move people who are unable to assist. It has a frame and a large sling to move the person. Before using it, ensure that you have been taught how to position the sling under the person, how to attach the sling to the frame, and how to operate the lift. Never leave your family member unattended while suspended in the sling.

CONSIDER FOR A MOMENT . . .

Which of these devices

have you heard of?

MOVING SOMEONE IN BED

Moving someone up in bed

People often slide down toward the foot of the bed, especially if the head of bed is raised. One caregiver can move the person to the side of the bed or up to the head of the bed.

Ensure the head of the bed is as flat as possible so you do not have to move the person against gravity. Remove the pillow from under his head and place it in front of the headboard. This ensures the pillow will not get in the way during the move and will protect his head if he goes up too far. To prevent injury to the neck, instruct him to tuck his chin.

If the person can help, instruct her to bend her legs and position her feet flat against the bed. Put one arm under her neck and shoulders and the other under her thighs. On the count of three, shift your weight as you move her up in the bed.

If this method is not useful, move only one part of the person's body at a time. For example, the upper body can be moved, then the middle, then the lower. Move each part diagonally toward the head of the bed. Place your arms under each part or use the draw sheet. Shift your weight.

If your family member is unable to assist, it is always desirable to have two people move him. A draw sheet can be placed under him. His arms should be placed on his chest. The two movers stand on either side of him and grasp the sheet. The sheet should be rolled so it is grasped as close to his body as possible. This will make the move easier.

If a draw sheet is not being used, two people can grab each other's forearms under the person's shoulders and thighs. Both people then shift their weight on the count of three.

A mechanical lift can also be used to safely move the person in bed.

Moving someone to the side of the bed

If your family member is to be moved to the side of the bed, place your arms under one part of him and move that part. You can also use a draw sheet.

If he can assist, have him move his buttocks, followed by his feet, and then his upper body. Assist him by shifting your weight from the foot closer to the bed to the back foot.

Two people can also move the person by standing on the same side of the bed. One person moves the upper body and the other moves the lower part.

Remember: Never reach over a side rail to provide care (overreaching).

Assisting someone to a sitting position

It is easier to assist a person into a sitting position on the edge of the bed if the head of the bed can be elevated. The person is almost in a sitting position just by raising the head of the bed. Then the caregiver only has to help the person to move her legs over the side of the bed.

To do this, move the person's legs and feet as close to the edge of the bed as possible. Use one hand to move the legs over the side of the bed while the other hand pushes up on the person's shoulder. Your hand on her shoulder not only helps her to sit up, it also provides reassurance to her and ensures that she does not fall forward or backward.

If the head of the bed cannot be elevated, assist your loved one to sit up. First, roll him onto his side. Assist him to sit up as he uses his arms to push up into a sitting position. His legs are moved over the side of the bed as he sits up. The amount of assistance you provide will depend on the amount of strength he has.

MOVING SOMEONE FROM BED TO CHAIR

Moving people from the bed to the chair stimulates them physically and mentally. It can also encourage them to become more independent.

If the person can bear weight, she should be able to stand and then be assisted into the chair.

There are several things to remember when moving your family member from the bed to the chair:

- Have him move towards his stronger side. He will be able to stand better on the stronger side.

- Ensure he has proper footwear to prevent slipping. Always use shoes or supportive slippers with non-skid soles.

- If transferring to a wheelchair, raise the footrests before the transfer and then return them to their usual position once the person is safely seated. This gets the footrests out of the way so he does not trip over them.

- Have the chair positioned close to the bed.

- Ensure the bed is at the lowest level possible to help the person to get in and out of the bed easily.

- Raising the head of the bed before assisting the person to dangle or stand will help with the move.

This decreases the amount of energy that will be required during the actual move.

• When the person has had a chance to dangle, assist her to stand. Position her feet apart and lean her forward slightly, as you would naturally do to stand from a seated position. Her feet should be flat on the floor. Facing her, place your hands around her waist or grasp the transfer belt. Let her put her hands lightly around your waist. Or, she can use her arms to push off from the bed.

• Use the rock and pull method to assist the person into the standing position. Instruct her to rock forward on each count and to stand on the count of three. Assist with this rocking movement by shifting your weight from the foot nearer the bed to the back foot. Repeat this weight shift with each rocking motion. The rocking will help build up power and momentum so it is easier for your loved one to stand.

• By placing your knee against her knee and your foot against her foot, you can provide extra support. On the third rock, pull her into a standing position.

- While holding the person, pivot so she is positioned in front of the chair. She should grasp the arm of the chair with a hand. Flex your knees and assist her to lower into the chair.

- Instruct your family member to let you know if dizziness occurs during the transfer. If she does faint during the transfer, do not attempt to hold her up. Instead, lower her to the floor as gently as possible. Be sure to protect her head. If she is unable to assist with the move, or can only help a little, a mechanical lift can be used to safely move her from the bed to the chair.

CONSIDER FOR A MOMENT . . .

What technique do you use to move
the person into a chair? Are you doing
anything that might injure your back?

MOVING SOMEONE FROM BED
TO STRETCHER

There will be occasions when your loved one will need to be moved from the bed to the stretcher. Normally, professional health care workers will perform this transfer but it is worth noting the tips and procedures in case you are involved. In addition to following the general principles for transferring, remember the following:

• Position the stretcher beside the bed.

• Ensure the bed and the stretcher are the same height.

• Ensure the brakes are on the stretcher and the bed.

• Always have a person stand on one side of the bed, while another stands on the opposite side of the stretcher. This is for your loved one's safety in case the bed or stretcher slips during the transfer, despite the brakes.

• If the family member can assist with the transfer, instruct him to move his feet, then his buttocks and finally his upper body to the stretcher.

- If he cannot assist, use a draw sheet under him. Cross his arms across his chest. Ideally, two caregivers will stand on one side of the stretcher and two caregivers will stand on the other side of the bed. A fifth caregiver will stand at the foot of the bed to move the person's feet. On the count of three, the person is moved to the side of the bed. (Use the same technique as discussed in the previous section Moving someone to the side of the bed). On another move, the person is moved to the stretcher.

- Make sure the person's body is centered on the stretcher.

- Make sure he is comfortable and raise the head of the stretcher.

- Advise him to keep his hands inside the stretcher to prevent bumping against doorframes during transport.

- If you are not able to position the stretcher near the bed, three people will be needed to move the person. Each person takes responsibility for one part - one takes the head and shoulders, one takes the hips, and one takes the thighs and legs. On the count of three, roll the person towards your chest and move as a unit to carry the person to the stretcher.

- If the person is large and dependent or if there are not enough movers, a mechanical lift can also be used to move him from the bed to the stretcher.

MOVING SOMEONE IN A
HOMECARE SITUATION

There are some special challenges to think about when you are caring for someone in his or her own home:

- There may not be another caregiver available to help you.

- You may not have any special equipment.

- You may not be able to raise or lower beds.

- You may be working in a small area.

- You may have to be creative as you plan your move. However, you must still make sure that the way you move the person is safe. Follow the guidelines for keeping your back safe. The surroundings should be as safe as possible. For example, the area should be well lit with an uncluttered path that is not slippery.

CASE EXAMPLE
MRS. GIOVANNI'S SITUATION

You are alone with Mrs. Giovanni who is in bed. She is weak on her left side. You are about to position her so she can eat her lunch. She is in a hospital bed and does not want to get out of the bed until later. You notice that she has slid down toward the foot of the bed. Transfer equipment is not available.

What position would be best? Describe the technique you would use to reposition her.

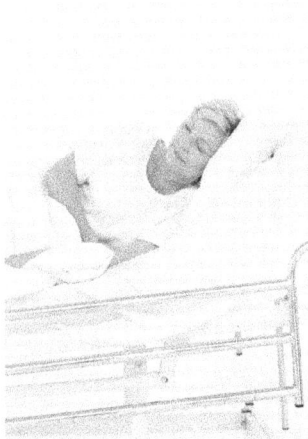

YOUR ANSWERS TO CASE EXAMPLE

SUGGESTED ANSWERS

Immediate priorities:

The best position for Mrs. Giovanni to eat her lunch is to be sitting up in bed. However, you must first move her up in the bed. You should:

Assess Mrs. Giovanni and her surroundings

You can then plan the move safely and ensure the environment is safe - uncluttered, well lit, etc.

Explain what you are about to do.

Provide Mrs. Giovanni with information so she can cooperate.

Adjust the bed.

Lower the head of the bed. (So you will not be moving against gravity.)

Lower only the side rail on your side of the bed.

Remove the pillow from under her head and place it in front of the headboard. (This ensures the pillow will not get in the way during the move and will protect her head if she goes up too far.)

Instruct her:

To tuck her chin. (This prevents injury to her neck.)

To bend her legs with her feet flat against the bed.

(This is the best position for her to be able to push with the legs.)

To push with her legs. Coordinate the move with Mrs. Giovanni by counting to three.

Assist Mrs. Giovanni:

To move with one arm under her legs and one arm under her neck.

Safety:

Follow the guidelines for keeping your back safe.

Weight shift during the move. To do this, you should have all your weight on the foot closest to the foot of the bed. As you move her, shift your weight to the other foot. This reduces the force needed to move her.

Comfort:

Raise the head of the bed and make Mrs. Giovanni comfortable.

CONCLUSION

Always use proper techniques to safely move your loved one. Ensure that you follow the advice of your health care professional or health worker.

Transferring someone without injury either to the person or to the caregiver is always the main priority.

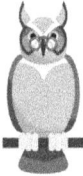

CHECK YOUR KNOWLEDGE

1. What factors can contribute to back pain in caregivers?
2. What should you assess before moving someone?
3. Define dangling. What is the purpose of dangling?
4. List 5 general principles for transferring people.
5. How would you transfer someone from the bed to the chair?
6. How would you move someone up in the bed if you were alone?
7. Describe how you would transfer someone to a stretcher if you could not position the stretcher by the bed.

TEST YOURSELF

Please circle to indicate the best answer:

1. You are moving someone to a stretcher. The person is able to assist. Is this a lift or a transfer?

a. Lift

b. Transfer

2. Mechanical lifts are a safe way to move a large person.

a. True

b. False

3. Raise the head of the bed before moving a person up in bed.

a. True

b. False

4. What is a trapeze?

a. A sheet under the person.

b. A belt around a person's waist.

c. A board between the bed and the chair.

d. A bar that hangs over the person's bed.

5. You are turning your body without twisting your back. What is this called?

a. Dangling

b. Flexing

c. Pivoting

d. Weight shifting

6. It is usually easier to tell the person not to assist with the move.

a. True

b. False

7. There can be special challenges when moving people in their homes.

a. True

b. False

ANSWERS:

1. b. This is a transfer. The difference between a transfer and a lift is that the person assists with a transfer, but not with a lift.

2. a. True. A mechanical lift is a safe way to move people who are unable to assist.

3. b. False. Ensure the head of the bed is as flat as possible so you do not have to move the person against gravity.

4. d. The overhead bar, or trapeze, is attached to the bed frame. It hangs over the person's upper body. The person grabs this bar to assist with moving in bed.

5. c. Pivoting is a technique used to turn the body without twisting the spine.

6. b. False. Encourage the person to assist as much as possible. Give him or her simple, easy directions throughout the transfer.

7. a. True. There may not be another caregiver available to help you. You may not have any special equipment. You may not be able to raise or lower the bed and you may be working in a small area.

REFERENCES

Butrej, T. (1998). Health & safety update. Responsibilities vs. rights: nursing uncooperative patients. Lamp, 55(11), 31-2.

Butrej, T. (1999). Repositioning a person in a wheelchair. Lamp, 56(5), 33.

Du Gas, B. W., Esson, L., & Ronaldson, S. E. (1999). Nursing foundations: A Canadian perspective (2nd ed.) (pp. 925-936). Scarborough, ON: Prentice Hall Canada.

Elkin, M. K., Perry, A. G., & Potter, P. A. (1999). Nursing interventions & clinical skills (2nd ed.) (pp. 76-81, 100-116). St. Louis: Mosby.

Kozier, B., Erb, G., Berman, A. J., & Burke, K. (2000). Fundamentals of nursing: Concepts, process, and practice (6th ed.) (pp. 1026-1029, 1035-1045). Upper Saddle River, NJ: Prentice Hall Health.

Occupational Safety and Health Administration U.S. Department of Labor [OSHA]. (2001). Nursing home for long term care, rehabilitation services. Excerpts from OSHA Ergonomic Report (sc940324) [Online]. Retrieved October 8, 2001 from: http://www.oshaslc.gov/SLTC/ergonomics/ergonomicreports_pub/fetysc940324.html

Owen, B. D. (1999, May). Preventing back injuries. American Journal of Nursing [Online]. Retrieved October 8, 2001 from: http://www.nursingworld.org/ajn/1999/may/heal059c.htm

Owen, B. D. (2000a). Teaching students safer methods of client transfer. Nurse Educator, 25(6), 288-293.

Owen, B. D. (2000b). Preventing injuries: Using an ergonomic approach. AORN Journal, 72(6), 1031-1036.

Potter, P., & Perry, A. (2001). Canadian fundamentals of nursing (2nd ed.). Ross-Kerr, J., & Wood, M. J. (Canadian editors) (pp. 1524-1536). St. Louis: Mosby.

Sinha, S. (1997). Words of wisdom from 500 great lives. Edmonton, AB: SKS Publishing.

Taylor, C, Lillis, C., & LeMone, P. (2001). Fundamentals of nursing: The art & science of nursing care (4th ed.) (pp. 984-995). Philadelphia: Lippincott.